# Daddy's

## Little

# Ballerina

## By
## Alicia Humphries

# Copyright

# CONTENTS

# A Word From Your Author

This is a work of fiction all characters are fictitious. Any similarity to any person or persons either living or deceased is purely coincidental.

Alicia Humphries writes erotic fiction encompassing taboo subjects. She sincerely hopes you find her work entertaining.

If that is indeed the case then please visit the site you download or purchased this book from and leave a review.

For further titles by Alicia visit my Author Page at Amazon.

Many Thanks

## Alicia xxx

# Daddy's
## Little
# Ballerina

## ON STAGE

My step dad new nothing about ballet, which is my passion but never the less he did everything he could to help me, taking me to dance classes and auditions nearly every day of the week, it seemed upside down.

My mother showed no interest in my dancing or indeed in her husband, in fact she was away on business yet again this time for two whole weeks.

I don't care too much, I'd rather spend time with Chris anyway, he'd been my step dad since I was twelve and now just four weeks after my eighteenth birthday he was more important to me than ever.

Important in more ways than one, you see I love my step father in ways that I really shouldn't, I can't remember when it first occurred to me but lately the feelings had been growing and growing. Lately whenever he was around my heart had beaten faster and my breathing had become a bit more difficult.

A week ago things came to a head when I'd woken up sweating from the best dream, I'd dreamt that he was in my bed touching me, I'd put my hands between my legs and felt the extra wetness there.

Since that night I'd been touching myself thinking about him every time I'd gone to bed and when he'd watched me dance I just seemed to have performed better and better. I knew it was silly he'd never be interested in me. After all he'd chosen my mum so it was obvious what his 'type' is.

She is tall dark haired with huge breasts. I am the

exact opposite. I'm tiny, short enough to be taken for a schoolgirl, I have no breasts whatsoever and I'm really skinny with blonde hair, a perfect ballerina physique.

I stop thinking all my thoughts as I take to the stage. An individual competition, I dance my heart out, I don't care about the hundreds of people in the audience or the judges, I only care hat Chris is watching me.

# THE DRESSING ROOM

I take my bow and head off into the wings with the other performers. Chris has come around and is there waiting for me, I smile up at him, I see a look in his eyes that I've not seen before, well not from him anyway, I ignore it shaking my head slightly trying to push the thought away but it won't go, the look was the same one I'd seen in Craig's eyes. The night I let him take my virginity.

We all march back on stage at the end of the competition and wait for the result.

When it is announced that I've won I can hardly believe it. The trophy, the flowers and the prize money all mine.

After the applause I walk off to the side of the stage again, but my Dad has gone.

The stage hand tells me he'd left a message that he'd be back in twenty minutes.

As usual at these events everyone dissipates really

quickly and after not very long I am standing backstage on my own.

The stage hand comes up to me, you can wait in there if you like, he points at a dressing room with a star on the door.

'Your dad will be back in a while but I have to leave, will you throw the latch when you go?'

'Sure' I tell him, why not, it's my local theatre, and everyone knows me.

'I'll leave a note on the stage door letting him know where you are.' He said before leaving.

Strange really I should be a bit spooked in the old theatre all by myself but I'm not, I'm still buzzing from winning the competition.

I go into the dressing room, it's a smallish room with its own shower room. I decide to have a quick shower before dad gets back.

It's so good to feel the water sprinkling across my

body, it's been a long day and I feel grubby. I turn off the shower and step out of the cubical, "SHIT!" I'd forgotten to check before I went in, no towels!

I step back into the dressing room and stop dead Chris is standing there, holding a huge bunch of flowers up in front of his chest.

I look past him at the hanger on the back of the door where the towel hangs but I don't move towards it. I stand letting his eyes sweep up and down me that look in them again.

He doesn't move either, he doesn't look away he just looks.

After what seems like forever he whispers, 'beautiful'.

My heart jumps, I can see myself in the huge dressing mirror surrounded completely with bulbs, It brings me back from the dream state I am in, and I cover my nonexistent tits with one arm and put a hand in front of my slit, suddenly aware that I am completely bald down there and that he can see my slit and my puffy pink clit which always protrudes slightly.

He speaks again this time to me instead of himself, 'you look fabulous princess.'

I feel my nipples harden and push against the inside of my forearm. Slowly I let my arm slip away from my tits and down to my side.

I keep my hand in front of my pussy my two middle fingers resting on my swelling clit, I feel my own pulse against the fingers.

He licks his lips, I feel myself getting hotter and damper between my legs.

The two of us have been standing completely still, there should be embarrassment and awkwardness but there isn't, I just feet horny and I can feel him radiating the same arousal too.

I smile at him and pull my hand up slowly revealing my slit bit by bit.

He looks down watching my every move. He places the flowers on the dresser, and moves towards me, as he stands towering over me I turn half sideways on and he puts his arms around me.

'Oh Chris' I said to him, 'you've no idea...'

'Hush there princess, I've been getting the vibe for a long while I've just been fighting it.' Then he leans down to me and kisses me full on the lips twisting me towards him at the same time.

His hand sinks straight down to where mine had been, his much bigger than mine he cups my pussy, the heat searing off him, sending the chill through my spine, I shiver, half from his touch and half from the water starting to evaporate off my body.

He takes his lips off mine he doesn't move his hand though, 'is this what you really want?'

It's all I can do to nod, understanding fully the implications of our so far unspoken agreement.

His eyes darken, 'take my cock out' he says in a

deep sort of soulful voice that dampens me even more.

I fumble both hands to his trouser front find his zip and pull it down.

I can feel myself going from timid hopefully to ravaging sex starved whore and the realisation drove me crazy, Chris wants me as much as I want him!

Oh yes, I'm not going to waste this opportunity it might never happen again, as I unbutton his trousers he pushes a finger between my legs to my pussy entrance,.

I grab each side of the now half open waistband and pull them apart as far as I can, then he pushes a finger into me, making me instantly feel feint, I groan but I kept my head down, sliding my hands around his ass and easing the trousers down a bit.

His cock springs into view I smirk to myself pull both hands back around and grab it with both of them.

His turn to make a sound as he pushes a finger into me deep, curling finding my 'G' spot sending vibrations through me.

Unlike Craig who'd used his finger just to lube me up before unceremoniously fucking me, dad wants to please me which makes me want to please him back.

He kisses me again his finger working magic inside me, I pull at his cock with both my hands rolling the skin back and forward over his moist head.

His hips move in and out with my hand and mine move in time with his thrusting too.

I have to break away from his lips I can't get enough air through my nose to keep up with the orgasm as it builds in every fibre of my being. I am surprised by the speed and violence that my feelings overtake me but as I am about to release myself onto his insistent and expert finger a hot sticky bullet hits me just under my tits at the top of my stomach.

He pushes his face into the top of my head and howls as he comes all over the front of me, it is so wonderful and unexpected his finger stills as his ass rams forward with each fluid filled pulse, five six seven times his hot jiz splashes on my stomach, before his movement calmed.

He takes a huge breath and starts to finger me again, his jiz running down my front slow and sticky.

He seems to be concentrating even more on pleasuring me he pushes his thumb between my slit and rims my clit as well as my inner front wall, I exploded for him, his finger movements changing pace to keep time with my own convulsions. I scream and throw my face into his chest as I come over and over.

When the climax eases so too does his frigging.

My hips rocking back and forth with his finger I don't want him to stop, and as if by some intuition he carries on, massaging me inside and out my body carries on with him and the climax builds again.

I come this time harder than before, he makes some grunting pain filled sounds, I realise I'm squeezing the hell out of his cock, he didn't complain, he just finger fucked me more.

I ease the pressure on his cock, he gasps. 'I'm sorry Chris' I say.

'Don't be,' he replies taking his hand from between my legs grabbing me under my ass and lifting me off the floor spinning to his left and sitting me down on the dressing table, I open my legs and he slides between them, his trousers now around his ankles, his shirt covered his cock which pushes out towards me like a teepee.

He lifts my legs by the back of my knees then slides his hands along my calves to my ankles, he carries on pushing up so that my feet point to the ceiling up by his shoulders he let go and my heels fall against his shoulder blades and he slips his hands under my ass again his thumbs prizing me apart. I feel the cool air across the inside of my slit as I open up.

I look down as he pushes into me, I let my head roll back as he forces his way in deep and firm.

I let out a long moan, 'oh Chris yes I've waited for this for so long.'

He pushes in and out building his pace as he grunts. I move my body forward pushing my head against his chest between my own feet put my arms around the outside of my legs and under his arms, I am completely doubled up he stands still cupping my ass and pushed me back and forward on and off his cock.

His shirt is getting wet from my mouth, not very lady like drooling but I can't help myself, 'yes Chris fuck me'. He grunts and throws my little body back and forth harder.

'Yes dad do it to me hard,' he increased the pace more, 'oh god Daddy fuck me,' the sound of me calling him Daddy seemed to drive him wild.

He rams me onto him so hard, the slapping and squelching sounds so loud they fill the room.

He is growling like some horror movie beast, my world fades from grey to black, under my eyelids.

'Fuck me daddy,' again the word makes him make even more effort, my little body begins to shake, not just the flesh rippling as I hit down against him but from the inside out, a shivering that seems to reach every part of me even my fingers and toes become slightly numb.

'You are so bendy princess, even more supple than you look when you dance.' I know what he means, being double jointed is a big plus for a ballerina and it seems for getting a deep fuck too.

I know there aren't many girls out there that can double themselves over like this, giving absolute access to an invading cock.

I giggle to myself, I don't mean to, it sort of forces its way out between my lips, I am clenching my teeth as my pussy clenches onto him our flesh seeming to become one inside me, I felt the juice flood down my tunnel covering his cock all around, he feels it too.

'Oh princess yes come for me,' he says I scream this time not able to control myself, 'yes daddy I'm coming, I'm coming,' again the sound of me calling him Daddy seems to help him find another gear.

He grinds up into me as he forces me down on him, finding new depths, which makes the climax take on a new dimension too. He slows with me as my orgasm subsides he rides me down off the crest.

I squeeze my arms around him, it feels like I am giving a thank you hug but I don't car, after all I am grateful to him. He'd found places and feelings in me I only dreamed existed.

He sits me back down on the dressing table and pulls out of me slowly and deliberately.

My legs flop down and dangle off the edge as he steps back.

He bends down pushes his trousers off and then stands in front of me removing his shirt.

Naked standing in the small room with me he looks

perfect, I can't help but look down at his lovely stiff cock, all wet and glistening with my juice.

My own stomach still has a large smear of his cum on it mostly dry now and cracking like a mud pack from my movements.

He moves back to me, I think he had just wanted to look at me.

I think he is going to push into me again, my pussy glowing in anticipation of more of his pummeling, but as he steps forward he kneels down on one knee pushes my legs up and apart across the top of the dressing table forcing the makeup and tissue boxes over, most of the aerosols and bottles already on their side having fallen over during his first fucking.

He moves to one side and kisses the inside of my knee sending pleasure waves through me, then he kisses down slowly inching towards my cunt, I gasp over and over again the closer he gets, but he stops short of my spread lips, he dusts across me breathing hot air onto my swollen clit then breathing in slow and deep letting out a satisfied guttural moan as he does.

He sweeps up to my other knee and repeats the soft slow kissing driving me completely to distraction.

This time when he reaches my opening he stills and blows gently onto the hood of my clit, I draw breath, another electric shock springs up my body.

He huffs a smile I look at my wide open pussy my inner folds swollen more than I'd ever seen them before.

He made no move, I sit here on the table, my legs completely split across the surface.

In the end I can't take it any longer, I was about to beg him when he spoke.

'You smell so sweet princess.'

'Oh daddy' my words escaping me in a long sigh my whole upper body melting.

'I want to taste you!' he continued.

My heart jumps and my stomach tightens at the sound of his words.

'Do you want Daddy to eat your pussy princess?'

I nodded

'I can't hear you?' he teased.

'Yes!' again words escaped me breathlessly.

'Still can't hear you princess!'

I know what he wants I put my hands delicately on the side of his head and push my fingers into his hair. 'Yes Daddy! I want you to lick me, I want my Daddy to eat my pussy.'

That's it. He drives his mouth straight onto me, taking the whole of my sex in his mouth, he applies some sucking pleasure, my ass moves backwards away from him e moves with me letting me know he has no intention of stopping.

The wet warm mouth is so new and so wonderful I don't know what to do I want to squirm but I don't want to move and risk changing the feeling, then my mind goes blank, his tongue pushes into the very hood of my clit, the bit that I had found myself numerous times when I'd played with myself, how does he know the exact point, actually I don't care.

He prods, pokes and swirls his tongue around bringing me to the edge of heaven in seconds, then he blows my mind, I would never be the same again I know.

Without warning or ceremony he pushes a finger into my ass hole, hard and true right up to his knuckle, I gush and squeal like a baby pig, for the first time I actual squirt, my hot fluid warming me as it passes down from my stomach along my tunnel and out into his mouth,

He gulps me down suckered onto my aching pussy.

'Daddy!' I scream, he makes humming sounds sending vibrations into me making the orgasm so deep, a second wave flows across me, more juice gushes from me , so much that he has to break away for a second.

My vision is actually blurred I couldn't have known what he would be able to do to me.

He half stands far enough to kiss me, I can smell my sex on him then I taste myself in the kiss, I'd once tasted myself but only a tiny tentative taste and that was before I'd frigged myself.

Now the taste is overwhelming my mind races, it is so filthy and dirty and yet so right. I lap around in his mouth searching out as much of myself as I can get my tongue to.

All around his mouth is wet I pull off the kiss and lick my cum off his face, having tiny little climax explosions in my stomach as I do.

'Dirty little princess,' he whispers in my ear.

I smile not wanting to stop licking my legs slowly coil back from being completely open, when I touch his legs with mine a thought springs into my head.

'I wonder what he tastes like?'

The thought gives me butterflies, then makes my stomach tighten and then it turns me on,

I stop wondering what it might taste like and know I have to know for sure, and I have to know right now.

'Stand up Daddy,' I murmur right by his ear.

'Knowing my intention he asks 'are you sure?'

'Yes' I say, 'I'm more than sure.'

'Have you done it before?'

'No Daddy.'

'Don't do anything you don't want to. He says meaning eating his juice I think.

'Stand up you dirty Daddy,' I speak playfully letting him know that I know my own mind.

His chest passes by my eyes then his stomach, 'IT' comes into view, I know already I would never get tired of seeing it. I slip my head forward and down, my hair brushing against him drawing a long sigh.

I take it in my little hands and squeeze, a tiny drop of precum comes out of the end like a welcome party.

My nerves almost get the better of me I take a deep breath to steady myself and then put my tongue out ever so slowly, I know my hot breath is washing across it his leg muscles flex and relax in jerky spasms.

I touch the end as lightly as I can, just enough to take the little drop off the tip. It's was pretty neutral tasting at first, I pull back and it makes a string between my tongue and his cock.

I move back in open my mouth, realise I'm going to have to suck the clear cream off.

As my mouth goes over the end he jerk and moans It shocks me a tiny bit but the overriding feeling is joy knowing I'm pleasing him, I clamp my lips over the end and suck pulling the precum into my mouth, 'ah' there it is a slight salty taste, fireworks erupt in my mouth. I want more, I want the real thing.

I slowly tentatively slide my mouth down, I'm going slowly out of caution, but the effect tells me I am doing something he really likes, more precum immediately.

'I've got to tell you princess knowing this is your first blow job is really driving me crazy.' He says in slow stammering breathy tones.

Oh yes I think just what I want. I close my eyes and drive down so that the whole thing goes into my mouth and throat.

I gag and pull off brace myself and open wide again.

One thing that ballet has taught me is that anything worth having needs effort and that sometimes you have to push through pain and discomfort, also practice makes perfect.

I put a hand under his large hanging sack and push my head forward.

I gag again but only pull back about half way just enough to be able to swallow my eyes are watering so much I can't see anything so I don't bother opening them as I force him into my throat again.

This time my watering eyes get worse but I don't gag.

He is panting hard he sounds like a Doberman after a long walk.

'Oh princess I'm gonna cum, if you don't want it in your mouth now's the time.'

I pull off him, his cock twitching like some small dying corpse. I lick the end, he makes to put his hand on it, I brush it away, and speak in the most serious manner I ever have, 'no Daddy I want to drink you all up like you did to me!'

'Oh shit princes,' I can tell there wasn't much time left, 'fuck my face daddy!' I say as I pull his balls towards me. He rams his cock into me, the force sending it a tiny bit further down my throat than I'd been able to get it a moment ago.

Bang, bang he shoves into my throat I do a silent scream on it knowing the vibration would be real nice, I squeeze his balls and then, heaven,

His thighs tighten and he shouts at the top of his voice 'PRINCESS' filling my belly up with cream, I pull back after the first couple of jerks so I cn get a good lode of it in my mouth.

It is stronger tasting than the precum feeling the slimy salty jiz plastering my mouth makes me damp, I hum partly to pleasure him but mostly as a reflex to such a great event.

When I am sure his balls are empty I suck back real slow kissed the end of his cock. And smile up at him.

* * *

# BACK ON STAGE

We are in the empty theatre, just the house lights on, Daddy sitting on a chair right at the front of the stage,

I dance for him, a naked dance.

He claps when I finish and stands up, 'princess you're the best.'

I run across the stage jump up into his outstretched arms. I wrap my legs around him his lovely juicy cock nestles against my still soak cunt, I kiss him hard 'fuck me Daddy.'

'I don't have any protection princess,' his face scrunched up obviously wanting it as much as me but trying to resist the temptation. I pull myself up on his shoulders and sink down on his shaft.

We both gasp out loud as he enters me and I envelope him. He stumbles back and sits in the chair.

I bounce on him until he comes again shuddering into me, I carry on forcing animal like sounds out of him, when I come he hugs me so tight rocking me back and forward milking my body of all I had.

He stands and carries me then lay me on the floor still inside me.

Now he unleashes his experience on me, finding angles and rhythms in me sending me up into the fly.

Five cataclysmic orgasms he forces out of me, I actually weep during the fourth and fifth, I think I might need medical attention afterwards.

When he finally shoots his lovely jiz into me again I am as limp as a dishrag, completely exhausted and in a state of pure bliss.

'I'm going to do that to you every day from now on princess.'

'Oh yes Daddy,' I say before being scooped up taken back to the dressing room then taken home.

www.ingramcontent.com/pod-product-compliance
Lightning Source LLC
Chambersburg PA
CBHW070511290526
45790CB00003B/1194